C000006670

Diabetes Prevention

Other Books by Rivkah Roth DO DNM®

At Risk? Avoid Diabetes by Recognizing Early Risk—A Natural Medicine Approach

At Risk? Expanded Workbook

DIABETES-Series Little Books:

Risk of Diabetes

Low-Carb for Diabetes

Gluten-Free for Diabetes

Minerals for Diabetes

Spices for Diabetes

Teas for Diabetes

Visible Risks of Diabetes

Das Kochbuch aus Zuerich (in German)

Das Kochbuch aus dem Bernbiet (in German)

Diabetes Prevention

Not Like The Last Thirty Years

Rivkah Roth DO DNM®

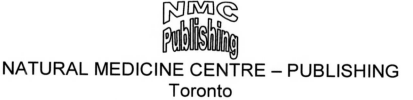

NATURAL MEDICINE CENTRE – PUBLISHING
Toronto

© 2009 by Rivkah Roth DO DNM®. All rights reserved.

No part of this book may be reproduced or transmitted in any form or by any means, electronic or mechanical, including photocopying, recording, or by any information storage and retrieval system, without permission in writing from the copyright owner.

Disclaimer

This book and its recommendations are not designed to replace a professional medical diagnosis and treatment.

It is the sole intent of the author to offer knowledge of a general nature and to create an understanding for the complex natural processes involved in metabolic diseases that may lead to pre-diabetes and diabetes. None of the information contained in this book is intended for diagnostic or treatment related purposes. The author and publisher disavow any responsibility for any decisions or actions with regards to and not limited to self-care, self-diagnosis, and self-prescription that you may want to undertake based on this book. The author and publisher strongly recommend that you seek medical help from your own licensed healthcare provider.

The statements and information in this book have not been evaluated by the American Food and Drug Administration (FDA) or by other National Health commissions.

Library and Archives Canada Cataloguing in Publication

Roth, Rivkah, 1950-
    Diabetes prevention : not like the last thirty years / Rivkah Roth.

ISBN 978-0-9812297-1-3

    1. Diabetes--Risk factors. 2. Diabetes--Prevention.
3. Diabetes--Popular works. I. Title.

RC660.4.R681 2009   616.4'62   C2009-903089-6

To order additional copies or volume orders of this book, contact:

 Natural Medicine Centre–Publishing
ISBN Paperback 978-0-9812297-1-3.
    "AvoidDiabetes"
www.avoidiabetes.com
nmcpublishing@ymail.com

For a Better Professional
and Public Understanding
of how to
Avoid and Prevent
Diabetes

Calls for proactive *Diabetes Prevention* grow louder.

Medical Diagnosis of diabetes on average is eight to fourteen years late.

Research has identified over fifty conditions that point to a *Future Risk of Diabetes*.

High *Socio-Economic Cost* is linked to exponential worldwide growth of *Diabetes Numbers.*

A predictable *Risk of Diabetes* is most closely connected with Westernized foods and lifestyle.

Diabetes numbers have risen at the same rate as *Grain-Carbohydrate Consumption* has increased.

Grain-Carbohydrate Addiction is real due to the presence of opioid exorphins in gluten amino acids.

About half of our population (close to 90% of South-Americans) carries a *Genetic Factor* (e.g. HLA-DQ2 or HLA-DQ8) that does not allow for grain-carbohydrate digestion.

Contents

A New Paradigm—Why Diabetes Prevention Must Start Long Before the Stage of Pre-Diabetes

Worldwide, patient numbers affected by diabetes and its complications[1] are escalating rapidly. Equally, the calls for diabetes prevention are growing.

However, diabetes numbers keep increasing even faster—a clear indication that the present preventive measures fail to show the desired results.

Patients considered "at risk" of developing diabetes—and targeted for prevention—are mostly those diagnosed with pre-diabetes or those with these serious conditions...

- ❑ overweight
- ❑ obese
- ❑ heart disease
- ❑ kidney disease.

Clearly, we must revise our assessment of "risk."

What if the main problem with effective diabetes prevention turned out to hinge on a mostly linguistic question? Namely, we need to better understand "risk" and arrive at a consensus on how to define "risk"?

---

1 IDF – International Diabetes Foundation numbers http://www.eatlas.idf.org/media

The Background

Diabetes is a metabolic disease. It has been known for over four thousand years and been written about since ancient Chinese medicine times.

For now, there is no cure for diabetes. It is generally acknowledged that it is mostly caused by diet and lifestyle and that it can be largely avoided or controlled, and occasionally reversed, by diet and lifestyle.

Recently, several public institutions, medical groups, and diabetes associations have started to call for earlier treatment and active "prevention" for those "at risk" of diabetes.

Most commonly, these are their suggestions:
- ❑ Develop concrete measures aimed at identifying those with pre-diabetes.
- ❑ Perform more frequent blood and urine testing[2].
- ❑ Postulate, for those identified as pre-diabetic, earlier and more aggressive medicating.

Missing the Mark

Unfortunately, defining pre-diabetes as the "at risk" stage for diabetes is clearly too narrow a classification.

A patient should not have to develop circulation disorders, vision problems, memory loss, and insulin resistance before being told that he or she is at risk of developing diabetes; in fact, that the patient "is now" pre-diabetic.

We all know that diabetes is a progressive and complex disease that leads to further complications. Worldwide, every ten seconds an individual dies from diabetes and related

2 For numbers see International Diabetes Foundation/IDF atlas: http://www.eatlas.idf.org/media

complications, while two individuals are newly diagnosed with diabetes[3].

According to the American Diabetes Association (ADA), of those born in the year 2000, one in three North-Americans and one in two minority individuals will develop diabetes later in life[4].

Already, fifty percent of those admitted to hospital emergency rooms after experiencing cardiovascular events are being diagnosed with diabetes at the time of their cardiac emergency.

The World Health Organization (WHO) writes "…taking into account deaths in which diabetes was a contributory condition, suggests that approximately 2.9 million deaths per year are attributable to diabetes[5]."

These numbers are shocking and present a rather sobering outlook. Quite obviously, we are missing the effective stage or mode of intervention.

Preventive measures are simply not effective when started in the last stages prior to a serious disease. Instead of targeting diabetes we must set our target prior to pre-diabetes.

So, wherein lays the problem?

Mainstream Diagnosis

What mainstream medicine considers the "early signs" of diabetes, the "Three P's" (*polyuria*, *polydipsia*, and *polyphagia*), in fact, already indicate that the patient has entered stages of function change.

---

3 http://www.idf.org/home/index.cfm?unode=3B96906B-C026-2FD3-87B73F80BC22682A

4 ADA website: Diabetes Statistics, The Dangerous Toll of Diabetes

http://www.diabetes.org/diabetes-statistics/dangerous-toll.jsp

5 WHO http://www.who.int/mediacentre/factsheets/fs312/en/

Most commonly, mainstream medicine writes a diagnosis of diabetes (see dark color segment in Figure 1) once blood sugar regulation no longer works and after initial function loss or cell damage have become serious issues.

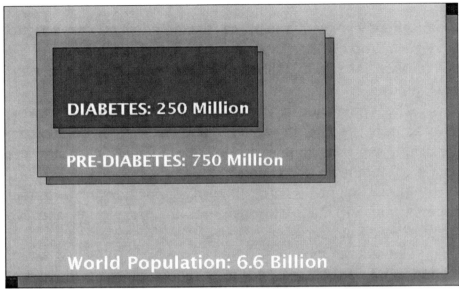

Figure 1 Mainstream Prevention Model; At Risk = Pre-Diabetes

Cell damage starts at blood sugar levels of 7mmol/L (126 mg/dL), the very threshold for a diagnosis of diabetes. To start checking for diabetes once the body has failed proper self-regulation is clearly a sign of "missing the mark."

Diabetes Diagnosis 8 to 14 Years Late

This approach to diagnosis leads to diabetes, on average, being diagnosed eight to fourteen years after the very initial signs surface.

Already in 2006, the participants at a Joslin Medical Centre Diabetes Conference were made aware of an eight to twelve year delay of diagnosis, and were reminded about the importance of capturing potential patients earlier.

Nothing has changed since then. More individuals are diagnosed at ever increasing rates—in their late stages.

But most worrisome is the fact that the numbers of overweight toddlers and teens skyrocket and that many of them are among the newly diagnosed diabetics.

Pre-Diabetes Diagnosis

As language indicates, before full-blown diabetes, the body passes a stage of "pre-"diabetes (see orange medium dark segment in Figure 1).

This stage of "pre-diabetes" is traditionally defined as "elevated blood sugar levels close to, but still below diabetic parameters."

At the time that a patient is diagnosed with pre-diabetes, the patient quite likely is already about six to eight years into the cycle mentioned above.

Pre-diabetes, thus, clearly is not the beginning of the disease and should not be considered the point at which to commence prevention.

However, linguistically, these patients are labeled as those "at risk of diabetes" when, in fact, they have long passed the at-risk stage and are well on their way to the full-blown disease (see Figure 1, Mainstream Prevention Model; At Risk = Pre-Diabetes).

This is the exact point where our entire understanding of prevention must undergo a dramatic shift. We must redefine "risk" as a point well prior to pre-diabetes.

Easier said than done—unless we manage to raise awareness that diabetes, on average, is diagnosed eight to fourteen years late.

Knowledge Transfer Barriers

Several years ago, the American Diabetes Association stated that pre-diabetes is a "serious" disease in its own right[6]. Yet, neither the ADA nor mainstream medicine as a whole act accordingly.

When you are ten minutes late for the train you still miss the train when you are six or eight minutes late. Why has this understanding still not made its way into medical offices and public awareness?

The facts are simple, straight and logical. Yet, with a headshake, we acknowledge that we are still told to prevent diabetes by concentrating our preventive efforts on those who have pre-diabetes.

Maybe we need to see this delay of information along the same lines as medical offices, TV commercials, and food reports still promote low-fat and high fiber diets[7] for diabetes avoidance when recent and credible research has concluded that "the right fats" and a "low-carb diet" stand a greater chance of regulating blood sugar levels.

Language as a Barrier

In order to communicate, we name things. This tool "word" or "name" that allows us to exchange knowledge also tends to block further thinking.

Once we call something by a name we tend to think within the box created by that name. Language judges and fixates by the choice of its words. A static approach does not make for change: change per definition is in motion.

---

6 American Diabetes Association http://www.diabetes.org/pre-diabetes/what-you-can-do.jsp

7 For instance all those "fiber" food TV ads.

The simple prefix "pre-" (before) in pre-diabetes indicates that this condition will take place "before" diabetes. Subconsciously, the brain concludes in a no-hurry, no-worry attitude, "okay, it is not diabetes yet... things, therefore, are still okay."

This approach of not taking "pre-"diabetes serious, entirely disregards the fact that diabetes is a progressive disease that does not start or get progressively worse only "after" its diagnosis (nor with a diagnosis of pre-diabetes) but long before.

Socioeconomic Impact

When people consume depleted, processed foods and drinks on a regular basis, their metabolism loses its ability to self-regulate.

When the body loses *homeostasis*, its ability to make up for imbalances and, especially, when it becomes nutritionally deprived, the likelihood of serious future illnesses grows.

Throughout history, growing incidence of metabolic illness surfaced at the height of many a civilization. Metabolic disease may have contributed to the downfall of history's legendary empires (China, Egypt, Rome).

For centuries, the loss of battle readiness seems to have coincided with the level of increased or perceived security and with greater acquired wealth.

Access to huge amounts of food and indulgence in many non-native foods were clearly associated with heart disease and diabetes problems. The Roman bucolic feasts are proverbial.

Why should it be any different today? Food and lifestyle still are number one contributor to metabolic disease.

Foods have Changed

No longer do we have access to fresh foods from the corner farm and our backyard. The implications for us are huge.

The further away from the natural state of our foods we move, the more likely becomes their impact on our human digestive system, a system that has changed little throughout millennia[8] of human development.

Loss of nutrients is a major factor in our agriculture of over-farming. In addition, when food requires to be transported to the consumer[9] over long distances, nutritional losses grow and toxic contamination levels increase.

For better storage and longer shelf-life, today we cultivate varieties that contain substantially more fiber, sodium, and nitrates than their equivalents sold a half a century ago.

At the same time, the desirable nutrient content of today's fruit and vegetables (calcium, other minerals and vitamins) is substantially lower and continues to drop.

We pride ourselves on our "easy lives" thanks to centralized mass production and worldwide availability of most foods—any time of the season.

A shift towards a healthier lifestyle might require a total rethinking of our work and living environments. The socio-economic impact of such a change away from processed foods to locally grown produce might, at least initially, produce a potentially devastating monetary effect on our economy.

This, quite obviously, raises the question, if such economic considerations play a role in the resistance towards a shift from our sick-care system to a true health-care and preventive approach.

---

8 USDA, Dietary assessment of major trends in the U.S. food consumption, 1970-2005

http://www.ers.usda.gov/Publications/EIB33/

9 University of Wisconsin, Department of Soil Science, Madison

http://www.soils.wisc.edu/~barak/poster_gallery/minneapolis2000a/index.html

Consumer Vulnerability

A change away from processed foods will most prominently impact on our big-time tax paying companies of the food industry, on big pharma, and even today's rapidly growing nutritional supplement industry.

What is good for the food industry, the pharmaceutical industry, or the media who get their advertising dollars and, lastly but not least, the tax-collecting authorities, is not necessarily good for the individual dealing with a health crisis.

Over the past several decades, this structure has lead to a clash between producers and consumers. The consumers pay fourfold:

- ❏ by buying the goods the producers and media want them to buy so they make more money,
- ❏ by lowering their immune system and getting ill due to eating nutritionally inferior, processed foods (literally, paying with his health),
- ❏ by losing income due to absenteeism or less efficient work (presenteeism), and
- ❏ by paying for more expensive sick-care and multiple medications (and possibly suffering early death).

However, to delay the necessary changeover to healthier lifestyles is not an ethical option. Such a delay would eventually defeat itself: people who operate below their physical and mental potential are inefficient workers. We already see a global increase in presenteeism and absenteeism rates. In the end, a sickly individual cannot efficiently contribute towards economic growth. Aside from the personal loss, such an individual costs the system dearly.

For exactly this reason, I believe that the present socioeconomic crises must be tied in with our failure to effectively maintain healthy, contributing individuals.

Cost Factors

Diabetes and its complications come at a high personal cost. Their financial, economic and social cost is exorbitant and ever increasing. The results of metabolic illnesses weigh heavily on the individual and the public purse[10].

Worldwide, 2007 spending estimates to "prevent and treat" diabetes and its complications stood at over 232 billion US dollars. Low estimates for 2025 call for more than 302.5 billion US dollars[11].

Already, the costs for employer health benefit contributions approach those for retirement benefits, and cost a North-American employer an untenable $8.74 per employee hour[12]. No wonder, many small businesses find these contributions unsustainable.

Health and Social Growth go Hand in Hand

What comes at a heavy personal price with unreasonable personal pain and sacrifice, unfortunately, represent a great economic stimulus. In 2007, USA's 24 million diabetics spent 174 billion US dollars in annual healthcare cost. This creates work in the pharmaceutical and health industries.

Also in the USA, lifetime medical treatment fees alone add up to $250,000 for every diabetic individual—in addition to diabetes prescription meds and drugs for diabetes complications. It, therefore, is not that likely that change is pushed forward from the top down. Even if it becomes equally

---

10 IDF – International Diabetes Foundation numbers http://www.eatlas.idf.org/media

11 IDF http://www.idf.org/home/index.cfm?unode=3B9691D3-C026-2FD3-87B7FA0B63432BA3

12 Employee Benefits Institute http://www.ebri.org/publications/facts/index.cfm?fa=fastFacts

unlikely that the affected individuals will be able to actively contribute to socioeconomic growth!

But consider this: due to sick days and untimely deaths, over the next ten years, the World Health Organization (WHO) estimates $555.7 billion in lost national revenue in China, $333.6 billion in India, $303.2 billion in the Russian Federation[13]...

Any new budget must include the factor of health and the need for disease prevention rather than focusing solely on remedying disease. Let us not forget that, especially with the aging of the baby-boomer, a slew of additional illnesses will enter the "must-medicate" stage already at and before the pre-diabetic stage.

Again, a definition of pre-diabetes as the at-risk threshold makes neither medical nor financial, nor social sense.

Society is Made Up by Individuals

Health may be elusive without an individual being willing to accept a strong measure of responsibility for his or her actions (smoking, alcohol consume, food choices, exercise habits, toxic surroundings, etc.).

Granted, not all diseases can be controlled, made better or made worse by lifestyle choices. But a large majority of diseases are directly tied to how we eat and live.

One thing is certain, personal irresponsibility when it comes to diet and lifestyle choices directly affects any foreseeable and broader economic downturn or recovery. Should we not start focusing on educational goals and on battling the information that nurtures and promotes the destructive habits?

---

13 WHO http://www.who.int/mediacentre/factsheets/fs312/en/

Public Stumbling Blocks

In summary, even if changing our eating habits would be easier than it appears to be, it is a highly disputed "hot iron." The changes that will drastically reduce our diabetes epidemic will need to affect every aspect of private, communal, political and economic life.

No wonder there is such a reluctance towards change!

Herein lays the problem. Our medical system is too overloaded and busy coping with those already too sick to turn their health around without serious medical intervention. Consequently, our medical system has neither time nor energy to absorb new knowledge over and above a new prescription recommendation for an existing condition.

"Not seeing the forest for the trees," becomes an unfortunate truth that suffocates any hope for effective change within the mores of the system.

There is little or no room left for learning to recognize that research already points to over fifty conditions that indicate a future risk of diabetes. Yet, the medical profession still considers these conditions as unrelated issues when, in fact, they should be largely understood as early stage metabolic problems and as parts of a whole instead of as a plethora of independent and unrelated states of dis-ease.

Consumer Mentality

The same goes for the patient. What we require is a major shift in the consumer mentality. Instead of "buying" what is being promoted (daily exposure to commercials and media opinion) we must learn to question and take responsibility for our individual health and wellness.

If we want to enable and empower a patient to take care of him or herself, obviously and foremost, we need to improve awareness levels and our lines of communication.

With our recently acquired deeper biochemical and bio-physiological understanding of metabolic diseases we should feel safe about not falling back into the fad-approach of the past three decades.

Newest knowledge and understanding, therefore, must be spread nationally and even on an international playing field—efficiently, in real time, not twenty or thirty years after the fact. And, valid reasons must be supplied along with bold suggestions.

In that sense, even research results must be questioned along with the "old wisdoms." Let us look at two recent examples:

Contradictive or Unclear Information

True to thorough and valid research and statistics, the American Diabetes Association confirms that "...the ethnic groups in the United States with the highest risk are African Americans, Mexican Americans, and Pima Indians[14]."

Just prior to that statement they claim that "...Americans and Europeans eat too much fat and too little carbohydrate and fiber, and they get too little exercise." No doubt they are correct about too much fat and too little exercise.

But, the ADA had started that very paragraph by saying that "...type 2 diabetes is common in people with these habits..." whereas, in the following paragraph, they postulate that "...people who live in areas that have not become

---

14 ADA Website http://www.diabetes.org/genetics.jsp

Westernized tend not to get type 2 diabetes, no matter how high their genetic risk."

Why then do we not draw logical conclusions? What really makes for Westernization? The answer is obvious: soda drinks and sandwiches, bagels, pizza, pasta and a slew of other grain-based, mostly wheat-derived processed foods most strongly stand for a Western diet. What these foods have in common are various forms of sugar, especially stemming from grain-carbohydrates.

We surely cannot claim that we eat "too little" carbohydrates—too little vegetable-source carbohydrates perhaps, but certainly not too little grain-derived carbohydrates.

Language and message are at odds here. The website gives the answer right there on that same page: stay away from Westernized food habits. Yet, that same leading national diabetes association recommends consuming more carbohydrates… Go figure!

Let us not forget this basic law: be specific or get misunderstood!

Incomplete Information

Now, for the second example: Research proves that, when it comes to blood sugar levels, a diet containing "whole grain" is better than one based on "white grain." Consequently, medical diet programs and diabetes associations advocate increased whole grain consumption. The "eat wholegrain" slogan is all over the media and advertisement pages.

More precise linguistics might carry the day. Slip in there the words "instead of" and the average consumer might stop eating an "extra slice" of whole bread toast just in order to consume that beloved cake flour cookie. Let us not forget that, in the end, this still counts as a "Westernized" high-carbohydrate food habit.

By the same token, research has yet to run adequate equivalent tests where a "whole grain" diet is compared to a "no grain" diet.

Neither has research sufficiently differentiated between those not able to digest grains[15] and the few populations doing well on grains.

We may not always have all the right answers, but we must learn to ask the right questions. If the industry does not do so, the consumer must learn to ask these questions and question the answers.

A New Approach to Education

Positive or negative, education holds the key. It is time that we use the health and food connection, not to sell more drinks, sugary juices, cereals, pizza and other processed foods, but to promote whole, unadulterated, unprocessed, fresh foods.

Changes may have far-reaching implications beyond our personal lifestyle to food-related businesses. New models for food production are called for and hold concurrent promise for carbon-footprint reduction (for instance by eliminating the need for long-distance food transports[16]).

We not only require individuals to restructure their approach towards health and food. New lifestyles can become part of the necessary approach towards greater health and disease prevention at the same time as they benefit a "greener" economy.

---

15 See same ADA web page http://www.diabetes.org/genetics.jsp

16 http://www.organicconsumers.org/

Telecommuting can easily go hand-in-hand with home-cooked meals prepared from locally produced, fresh and unprocessed ingredients and a healthy, environmentally conscious lifestyle.

But, while such new approaches become necessary for each individual, they have great implications on a greater socioeconomic level. Quite obviously, changes to city and community planning will become necessities.

Westernization is Not the Answer

Most importantly, we have to stop projecting on other populations an "it's only good if you copy us" attitude along with imposing our supposedly "developed" Western living style and food habits.

Rising rates of metabolic diseases have proven it: our Western approach to outsourced food preparation has proven to be destructive to human health and the environment and does simply not work.

Time to change and walk the talk!

The Underestimated Risk

Today, two to three times as many individuals have pre-diabetes than there are people with diabetes. This is a solid predictor of how our active diabetes numbers will continue to grow sharply over the course of the next six to ten years.

Since pre-diabetes clearly is not the beginning of the disease, and since we know that diabetes can be controlled (and perhaps avoided or reversed) largely by diet and lifestyle, it becomes mandatory that risk recognition of possible future diabetes start earlier—much earlier.

As we have mentioned earlier, research already points to well over fifty conditions that may indicate a possible risk of diabetes later in life (lightest color segment in Figure 2).

Truly, long before serious disease sets in, it is not the orange pre-diabetes segment but this "yellow segment" that represents the real "at risk" population.

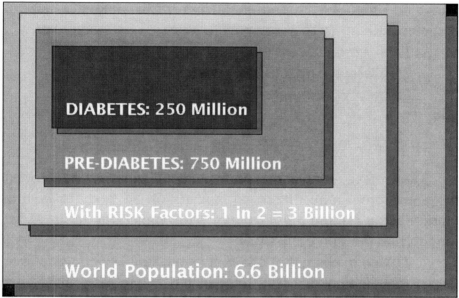

DIABETES: 250 Million

PRE-DIABETES: 750 Million

With RISK Factors: 1 in 2 = 3 Billion

World Population: 6.6 Billion

Figure 2 Newly Required Understanding of At Risk = >50% Population

The individuals who experience some of these over fifty conditions are the ones we need to address with the message that diabetes is largely avoidable. In "At Risk? Avoid Diabetes by Recognizing Early Risk—A Natural Medicine View" I describe and document the over fifty most obvious indicators identified to date by mainstream medical research[17].

---

17 See extensive bibliography and research article listing in "At Risk? Avoid Diabetes by Recognizing Early Risk—A Natural Medicine View" by Rivkah Roth DO DNM, ISBN 978-1-4257-6169-1

"Seeing" the Obvious

The public and the medical community must recognize that an individual occurrence of these fifty-some symptoms and conditions may not necessarily indicate a future risk of diabetes.

However, the repeat or simultaneous occurrence of three or four of these over fifty conditions, even if seemingly unrelated, may be strong indicators of a potential risk of diabetes later in life.

Take for instance a triad such as...

❑ bilateral carpal tunnel syndrome

❑ polycystic ovaries or erectile dysfunction,

and

❑ stress.

All these conditions, particularly if experienced around the same time, may reflect an inability of the body to control blood sugar-related processes. We must learn to start recognizing the true early signs.

Today, to claim that one in two individuals worldwide is at risk of developing diabetes later in life is probably already a conservative estimate—especially, when we add up all the many risk indicators. Now, if we add to this that diabetes shortens life expectancy by twelve years—just maybe—we will be seeing the urgency of the challenge.

A starting beer-belly and overweight alone already make for half of our population—never mind all those people potentially struggling with adrenal (stress) or other endocrine imbalances, sleep disorders, hypertension, and all the remaining fifty-some risk-indicating or predisposing conditions.

Along with the message that diet and lifestyle do largely determine personal health, we also must raise public awareness about the predictive ability of many of these over fifty risk indicator conditions. Clearly, medical education alone is not enough. The need for more specific education well beyond the medical community itself is more than evident.

Structures of Health Promotion

Growing diabetes numbers, along with worldwide doctor shortages, first and foremost necessitate an approach that stresses education and awareness about the importance of our eating habits, lifestyle, and food marketing patterns.

Unfortunately, that is exactly what we did in the 1980ies (in good faith) and what may have heavily contributed to our present metabolic health crisis.

Not long after we elevated the orange juice, cornflake, sugar, and milk breakfast to golden standard status, the troubles with diabetes started. So did increased numbers of infertility issues, polycystic ovary syndrome, many gastrointestinal problems, skin diseases, chronic pain conditions, such as fibromyalgia, and many more health problems.

Once again, we will need to explore ways to downstream not opinions and individual agendas, but proven working models based on solid biochemical reasoning and not solely on one or two (possibly elliptical) research trial. Clearly, mainstream medicine needs to continue focusing on their "sick care approach" and look after those already sick: the pre-diabetics and the diabetics.

But, we need a true health promotion approach to directly address the individuals possibly at risk—not simply those with pre-diabetes. The natural medicine system can become such an educational tool, and so could be, with some modicum of consensus, a new arm of government, media, public institutions, schools, even food producers and retailers, city planners and architects[18].

Already we are quite clear on the "what" and the "that"—the "how" still presents a huge challenge.

Food for Human Health and Function

Nobody—emphasis on "no body"—puts diesel fuel into the gas tank of their gasoline-fuelled car and expects the car to work flawlessly. Yet, this is how at least half of our population nourishes their body by feeding it what it cannot break down. The outcome is entirely predictable: the human mechanism breaks down.

It is time that we recognize and acknowledge that the digestive system of a significant percentage of our world population is not equipped to handle (at least certain) grains. In many indigenous peoples these genetic traits (HLA-DQ2 or HLA-DQ8 and some others) surface in close to 90% of individuals. In the North-American population the rate stands slightly above 40%. Future recommendations, therefore, must take this genetic aspect into consideration.

No One-Size Fits All

For this above mentioned genetic reason the presently practiced one-size-fits-all approach is no longer adequate or acceptable.

In the following chapter, we will look in greater detail into this issue of genetic predisposition towards certain foods. The fact that such large population percentages are affected by a

---

18 http://www.healthycities.org/overview.html; http://www.euro.who.int/healthy-cities

genetically built-in food intolerance, certainly calls for a new approach to dietary measures.

We have all learned in our physiology and biochemistry classes that food determines how the body works. Yet, according to our media info and advertisement barrages, it supposedly is okay to feed the body the right foods rarely or only part of the time (once every blue moon) and the rest of the time to follow our desires and cravings.—Never mind that cravings and illnesses are our body's way of letting us know that it is lacking necessary nutrients and building elements.

A "little less" does not protect the body from negative effects. We "eat to live," and we "are what we eat."

Avoiding Diabetes—Naturally

The most interesting observation is that to "change diet and lifestyle" is the accepted medical recommendations for most of our over fifty diabetes risk indicator conditions. This approach offers an easy and cost-effective solution that does not require expensive drugs and treatments and could go a long way reducing our worldwide shortage of doctors.

Yet, surprisingly, few mainstream doctors do take food intake totally serious. Until someone is clearly sick, they rarely suggest food changes; and even then, most MDs prescribe medications because they have no time educating their patients, don't believe in the true impact of food, or do not feel that they can subject their patients to any radical changes.

Implementing food and lifestyle changes early, generally reduces or removes the triggers that otherwise might lead to a future with diabetes and a slew of other illnesses from hypertension to heart disease, kidney disease to blindness, or bad wound healing to the need for amputations. Nobody disputes these facts and the potential for change in our own hands.

In Summary

At the beginning of this section we asked: What if the main problem with effective diabetes prevention turned out to hinge on a mostly linguistic question, namely, "How do we define the stage of 'at risk'?"

We must stop talking about an individual as being "at risk of diabetes" once he or she is diagnosed with pre-diabetes. A person with pre-diabetes is already seriously sick.

Instead, we would do well to promote public awareness campaigns and advocate for "Early Risk Recognition and Avoidance" long before the estimated additional two billion people worldwide who are at risk and have not yet reached the pre-diabetic or diabetic stage become sick.

The Outlook

An approach of true prevention will necessitate:

1. A new definition of health, the "at risk" stage, and of disease.
2. A transdisciplinary approach to the changing values and opportunities.
3. A shift towards holding each individual responsible for healthier living.
4. Advocacy of an intimate familiarity with and knowledge of the at least fifty risk indicating symptoms, diseases and conditions.

5. An acknowledgement that, worldwide, certain genetic predispositions do not allow for the digestion of grains, and that these genes are present in large segments of our population putting them at risk of diabetes and other metabolic diseases.

6. A subsequent shift may be required away from our high and disproportionate grain and specifically wheat use along with the avoidance of other gluten grains and gluten-containing products.

The Expected Impact

At the same rate as we raise levels of health, this approach away from a grain-dependent culture is bound to impact on:

7. Food industry through the call for local production.

8. Farming by favoring smaller local producers and smaller, more diverse crops.

9. Pharmaceutical Industry by allowing it to refocus on genetic and traumatic diseases and those conditions requiring surgical intervention.

10. Cityscapes and community building aimed at micro-production of food.

11. Work environment changes that support tele-commuting and family-centric lifestyles.

In addition to fostering better health, all these changes will contribute to stress-reduction and a greener environment.

Risk Avoidance—Not All Foods are Beneficial

There are several contentious issues when it comes to avoiding the risk of diabetes. Consensus on the need for exercise is widespread. When it comes to diet choices, however, controversies flare up.

Comparative Research may be Relative

In many instances, we need to better define ranges. For instance, some dieticians define a low-carbohydrate diet as less than 50 grams of carbohydrates per meal, others as less than 50 grams per day, and those of us with extensive patient experience in the field, as less than 30 grams of grain-carbohydrates per day.

Another example: few diet studies prequalify participants as to their HLA type. Knowing what we know today, individuals of the HLA-DQ2 and DQ8 type may react to grain carbohydrates, sugars, and fibers very differently from individuals without that particular genetic heritage. Research trials, therefore, may have to become more population specific.

In the field of natural medicine we often prequalify certain results as to certain groups. Adopting such an approach for conventional medicine might make more sense too. Not considering these HLA types when enrolling study subjects in metabolism-related research may explain some of the huge differences between parallel trials or between practical results and a particular research outcome.

Most conventional research is relative and comparative. Among the first questions we should always ask is what the particular project does not compare with and, thereafter, what helps us understand possible reasons behind the results, and what further questions need to be asked and researched.

Recommendations Rarely Reflect Research

Despite these shortcomings, research has outlined the most effective dietary measures with regards to avoiding metabolic diseases and diabetes.

For instance, research now advocates a carbohydrate-controlled diet rather than the formerly proposed low-fat diet[19] for those suffering from metabolic disease.

Similarly, low-carbohydrate diets recently have been credited with better blood sugar control than high-fiber diets[20].

However, neither of these research projects questions possible associations and underlying issues, nor if the results "make sense." The "why" has become less important than the "what" or the "that."

For argument's sake, let us look at possible explanations of the present carbohydrate versus fat versus fiber controversy:

A low-fat diet may not allow for proper mineral and vitamin absorption in the duodenum and the jejunum (small intestine sections following the stomach). Neither does a high-

---

19 Nutr Metab (Lond). 2008 Dec 19;5:36

20 JAMA. 2008 Dec 17;300(23):2742-53

carbohydrate diet in those of HLA-DQ2 or HLA-DQ8 type allow for digestive absorption due to inflammation.

Similarly, keeping carbohydrates to those carbs not causing inflammation in the duodenum or other parts of the intestines keeps down inflammation and allows for better mineral and nutrient absorption.

On the other hand, while no doubt fiber is preferable to processed, fibreless mush, let us not forget that in today's vegetables and fruits fiber levels have increased by up to 1200 times[21].

At the same time, a negative response to fiber may be connected to the small intestinal duodenum being affected by inflammation. All these scenarios affect the research outcome but are generally neglected in the result reporting process.

Major diabetes associations and their journals have published these findings independently—mostly without drawing the necessary conclusions, however.

Medical information and public awareness still hugely lag behind without acknowledging what makes sense biochemically and physiologically.

Medical Prejudice

Since many individuals at risk of diabetes tend to be overweight, medical practitioners still widely recommend low-fat or fat-free diets.

This again happens to be a linguistic issue: The "fat" of an overweight person is not equal to the "fat" that same person consumes. Despite this knowledge we tend to forget that fat may not make fat, but grain carbohydrates do.

---

21 Pawlick, Thomas F., The End of Food: How the Food Industry is Destroying our Food Supply – and What you Can Do About it. Greystone Books, Canada. ISBN 978-1-55365-169-7

Unfortunately, we also encounter a significant level of prejudice among the medical community. Many doctors even refuse taking on "fat" patients. They anticipate these patients to remain "uncontrolled eaters" and not able to show health improvements.

Linguistic Simplification

We must pay greater attention to linguistic definitions and concepts; and it is time to look further. For instance, lack of portion control is rarely the cause of disease but the result of underlying issues.

If a practitioner suggests thyroid, adrenal, or other endocrine tests, or maybe states, "we must look closer at your cravings," you may be in good hands.

However, when a doctor categorically states, "you must lose weight," it generally indicates that the practitioner may have failed to understood the process of weight gain and the reasons behind a patient's risk of diabetes and their inability to control their appetite.

Such a practitioner is stuck in simplistic language-driven understandings. Everyday word use overrides the learned comprehension of logistic biochemical and biophysiological processes. Such a doctor's patient best looks for another doctor.

Isolating Problems vs. Integrating Problems

To remain with today's leading topic of obesity: Most overweight and obese patients already have a long history of failed diet attempts. Clearly, the answer to their issues must be sought somewhere else than simply by uttering a statement of "they are fat and out-of-control eaters."

Culprit stressors leading to obesity may vary from work, life, and relationship stress to environmental and food stress. Illness prevention—and diabetes prevention, specifically—thus, needs to be addressed in the context of a patient's daily life.

The medical community must be reminded that isolating problems and viewing diseases out of context can be no more than one working tool prior to seeing the bigger picture and integrating or relating problems.

Serious illness rarely comes alone. Learning to recognize illness complexes, therefore, is a must. For instance, today in many cases, the basis for nutrient deficiencies, cravings and, eventually, food addiction stems from the body's inability to process grains.

The Role of the Media

The message promoted to and by the media is no different. Most articles, interviews and media ads continue to push high-carbohydrate, high-fiber, and low-fat foods on those at risk of metabolic problems. They too miss the point: the "good fats" do not make the body fat, sugars and starches do.

Following basic nutrition concepts, advertisements reason that the body needs carbohydrates for energy. They forget that our green and colorful, non-starchy vegetables provide us with ample of those needed "good" carbohydrates.

They overlook that the worst of the sugars are converted from our highly publicized and advertised grain-carbohydrate based processed foods. They do not tell that, when it comes to grain starch being converted to sugar, there is no significant difference between whole grains or processed grains.

Again the public is left with a fuzzy linguistic understanding of "you are fine as long as you eat whole grains." In order to make a significant step towards diabetes prevention we need a different message.

Understanding the Issues

The vicious cycle is simple: excess grain-carbohydrates (whole grain or not) cause intestinal inflammation followed by nutrient malabsorption and mineral deficiencies.

The bottom line is that several of our nutrients and vitamins require dietary fats (the right ones) in order to be absorbed into the body. Eating fat-free but high-carb is simply not the answer to good health.

Why then do many diabetes diets and diabetes educators still recommend unreasonably high carbohydrate amounts? Just to sell more meds? Are we afraid to tell an individual that serious lifestyle and diet changes (not baby steps) are needed if they really want to turn their health around?

The Brutally Honest Truth

We must keep in mind: if the individual is one of those genetically unable to digest grains, chances are it will need to store the excess "sugars" in the body's fat tissue. No surprise that we are facing such a self-destructive obesity epidemic!

This happens if the body cannot burn off excess carbohydrates into energy…

❑ if the body does not produce sufficient amounts of insulin (*hypoinsulinism*).

❏ if the body has become resistant to the body's insulin (insulin resistance or *hyperinsulinism*)[22].
❏ if the person is of HLA-DQ2, DQ8 or another genetic type not able to handle certain grain carbohydrates.

Maybe, if the public were to understand this, it would be easier to convey messages about diet and lifestyle requirements for health.

Oxygen versus Carbon Dioxide

Grain (carbohydrates) play a significant role with regards to our ecosystem. Grain farming accounts for one of the highest carbon footprints. It presents a huge drain on energy consumption and adds to pollution due to the need for transporting and processing of raw materials and processed grain-based foods.

Grain carbohydrates also affect the human ecosystem:
❏ Excess carbs are stored in our fat cells.
❏ Fat cells keep out water.
❏ The more fat cells the body carries the less oxygen the body has available for its organs to function.
❏ The higher the number of fat cells, the lower the proportion of blood per pound of body weight.

This directly affects how much oxygen is available to the body: A healthy person on a balanced omnivore diet exhales 80 units of CO_2 for every 100 units of O_2 inhaled. This leaves the body 20% of oxygen to drive the necessary body functions (kidney, heart, brain, etc.).

On the other hand, an individual on a high-carbohydrate diet exhales up to 100 units of CO_2 for every 100 units inhaled.

---

22 Ann Med. 2006;38(6):389-402

This leaves the body none or little oxygen for healthy function and puts the body under oxidative stress. In response, inflammation spreads and metabolic processes develop.

Clearly, reducing the (grain-)carbohydrate intake has the ability to reduce the human CO_2 output[23] along with the resulting brain fog, lack of energy, intestinal problems, heart and kidney disease, or diabetes.

It stands to reason that reducing our grain consumption will add to better health—at least for those of HLA-DQ2 or DQ8 types.

Grain Carbohydrates Drive up Blood Sugar

It is clear that excess sugar causes havoc in those genetically so predisposed and not able to convert sugar. We know that starch-based carbohydrates in excess of 10 to 12 grams per meal tend to drive up blood sugars.

Blood sugar spikes nearly always lead to the feared blood sugar rollercoaster: A "high" is followed by a "low." Every low then tricks the liver into producing a "replacement sugar" (glycogen)—and the rollercoaster starts anew.

It simply makes no sense that so many diabetes diets still suggest carbohydrate intakes of 50 to 80 grams of starch-based carbohydrates per meal. This adds up to daily totals in excess of what a healthy and physically active body is able to burn off.

The bottom line is:

An individual at risk may achieve consistent blood sugar levels by keeping below a daily maximum of 30 grams of grain carbohydrates with the prevailing recommendation of…

- ❑ 6 grams maximum for breakfast and
- ❑ 12 grams each maximum for lunch and dinner.

---

23 Zhonghua Yi Xue Za Zhi (Taipei). 1996 Nov;58(5):359-65. J Nutr. 2007 Feb;137(2):363-7.

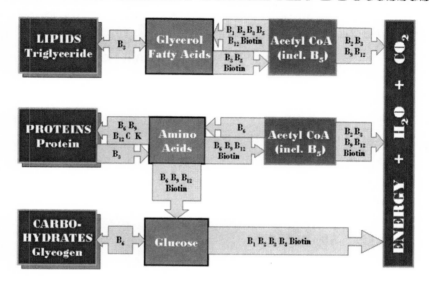

Figure 3 Fat, Protein and Carbohydrate Digestion Process

The Culprit Sugars

It does not only take sugar to make blood sugar and energy. Let us not forget that the body can convert fats and meat proteins to energy too. In fact, excess meat proteins get converted to sugar and are stored in the body's fat cells. This in turn jeopardizes proper hormone production.

Possible "sugar dangers" therefore, come in many forms:
- ❑ The extruded or manufactured "sweet stuff"
- ❑ The natural sugar in fruit
- ❑ The natural sugar in starchy vegetables

❑ The sugar converted from grain carbohydrates

❑ The sugar from anything ending in –ose.

With over 70%[24] of the world's population being lactose intolerant, the sugar converted from lactose (dairy products) is particularly contentious. One of the possible issues may be because of its casein-based opioid component (see gluten discussion).

It is simply not sufficient to avoid these "sweets." They all add to the influence of grain-carbohydrates on the human digestive system.

Ask any diabetic who regularly measures blood sugar values (no matter if type 1 or type 2 diabetes). They will confirm that eating any form of grain-carbohydrates and often also dairy products necessitates higher levels of medication to avoid blood sugar spikes and imbalances.

Excess Carbohydrates Affect Body pH

Sugar in any form (including grain carbs and lactose) turns the body acidic. Along with changes in the pH value this affects the body's electrolyte balance[25], immune system and regulating mechanisms. Tiredness, especially after meals, brain fog, forgetfulness, or lack of focus are unavoidable results and easily may serve as early risk indicators of diabetes.

We frequently forget that carbohydrate digestion starts in the mouth (versus protein digestion in the stomach, and fat digestion in the small intestines). Whenever we ingest foods that

---

24 Alimentary Pharmacology & Therapeutics Volume 29 Issue6, Pages 677 – 687; Published Online: 13 Nov 2008

25 Merck Manual http://www.merck.com/mmpe/sec12/ch157/ch157a.html

our body does not properly digest or that we are allergic or sensitive to, we develop gastro-intestinal issues.

Bloating, gas, loose stools and diarrhea or constipation, all are signs of gastrointestinal inflammation and may also serve as early indicators of a metabolic risk and future diabetes.

Carbohydrates Affect Human Digestion

Our present grain production is simply unreasonable. For instance, in the USA every single person on average consumes one kilogram of grain in one form or another per day[26] (from baked goods to grain-fed animal products).

Worldwide, for the last several decades, wheat has replaced traditional indigenous food sources and grains. During those same decades, the numbers of those affected by metabolic disease and diabetes have grown exponentially.

Late Addition of Grains to Human Evolution

It is important to remember that eating grains is a fairly recent addition to our human evolutionary development (latest 10,000 years of the 2.5 million years of hominoid development). This is simply not enough time for the human genetic make-up[27] to adapt to digesting grains.

Humans simply miss several enzymes necessary to digest grains. The best illustration for humans as hunter-gatherers comes from the fact that our young—like those of cats, dogs, and other carnivores—must be nurtured for months

---

26 http://www.fas.usda.gov/grain/circular/2009/01-09/graintoc.asp

27 Eur J Nutr. 2000 Apr;39(2):67-70.

and years before they can crawl, walk and eventually provide for themselves.

Eating and digesting grains comes natural only to true vegetarians (horses, deer, cows, elephants, and others), whose young ones are up and running within half an hour to an hour of birth.—I have yet to witness that human baby skipping out of the hospital delivery room while mamma is still being tended to delivering her afterbirth...

"Improved" Grains—The Gluten Connection

Grains are starches and, as such, are high in carbohydrates that raise blood sugar levels. But not all grains are alike.

Increasingly, we breed, grow, process, sell, and consume grains that have been selected for their improved storage ability and texture after processing. These traits are largely achieved by increasing the gluten content in those grains.

Gluten is a group of storage proteins present in some of our major grains and all their derivatives:
- ❑ Wheat
- ❑ Barley
- ❑ Rye
- ❑ Spelt
- ❑ Triticale
- ❑ Oats (due to contamination).

Through my clinical work, I have long suspected a strong link between gastro-intestinal inflammation, gluten-sensitivity and diabetes. Clinical results with a gluten-free diet for type 1 as well as type 2 diabetics have been promising.

Recent clinical and research data confirm the presence of shared genes between diabetics and those affected by celiac disease, a form of gluten-sensitivity[28].—The same research papers also mention the possibility of controlling and maybe reversing (at least) type 1 diabetes by following a gluten-free diet[29].

Quite recently, a 2008 continuous education seminar of the American Society of Health-System Pharmacists[30] run in conjunction with the National Foundation for Celiac Awareness postulated the prevalence of unconfirmed celiac disease in the USA as being ten times higher than the prevalence of type 1 diabetes.

How long will it be for the medical profession to start checking for the presence of gluten-sensitivity symptoms?[31] Diagnosis of celiac disease (the most severe form of gluten intolerance) on average takes 11 years. A simple DNA test could potentially spare years of agony, a slew of metabolic complications, and eventually diabetes.

Genetic Make-up and the Grain-Gluten Factor

Some of the most prominent of the genetic factors linking gluten-sensitivity and diabetes are the human leukocyte antigens…

❑ HLA-DQ2
❑ HLA-DQ8.

---

28 Med Hypotheses. 2008;70(6):1207-9. Epub 2008 Feb 4; J Clin Invest. 2006 Aug;116(8):2226-36. Epub 2006 Jul 27; J Autoimmun. 2008 Sep;31(2):160-5. Epub 2008 Aug 8; Diabetes. 2008 Sep;57(9):2348-59. Epub 2008 Jun 12.; N Engl J Med. 2008 Dec 25;359(26):2767-77. Epub 2008 Dec 10; Curr Opin Allergy Clin Immunol. 2007 Dec;7(6):468-74;
and countless other references.

29 J Clin Endocrinol Metab. 2003 Jan;88(1):162-5

30 American Society of Health-System Pharmacists http://www.ashp.org/

31 ASH: Common genes contribute to blood pressure regulation http://www.medpagetoday.com/14131

HLA-DQ2 is most common in individuals with roots in Western Europe, especially Spain and Ireland. It also occurs in North and West Africa, Central and Southeast Asia and China.

HLA-DQ8 is prominent in Hispanic populations (up to 90%; equal to their diabetes rates), indigenous Americans (in the 50% range), Asia, Thailand, Northern Europe, Russia, Scandinavia, Germany, France, British Isles, and several Bedouin populations[32].

With continuing research, new genetic factors and links are being identified. Meanwhile, HLA-DQ2 and DQ8 average over 43% in our North-American population. Without even including other risk factors, these two genetic traits alone already indicate a possible risk of future diabetes for one in two individuals worldwide.

With regards to our growing diabetes epidemic it is most important that we understand that celiac disease is only the most severe form of gluten intolerance or gluten-sensitive enteropathy, as it is also called. Unfortunately, gluten-sensitivity is rarely detected unless it leads to severe illness.

Many questions remain with regards to type 2 diabetes and a possible gluten connection. For now, most research points to a direct link between celiac disease and type 1 diabetes (particularly if combined with episodes of hypoglycemia).

So far, only minor references point to late onset diabetes[33]. Yet, abstaining from gluten grains appears to reduce gastrointestinal symptoms in many type 2 diabetics along with providing better blood sugar regulation.

---

32 Middleton D, Menchaca L, Rood H, Komerofsky R (2003). "New allele frequency database: http://www.allelefrequencies.net". Tissue Antigens 61 (5): 403-7. PMID 12753660. and http://en.wikipedia.org/wiki/HLA-DQ8 for over 60 citations

33 Arq Bras Endocrinol Metabol. 2008 Mar;52(2):315-21

A Different "Staff of Life"—Gluten Grains

Several of the shared HLA factors between diabetes and celiac disease may point to carbohydrate intolerance and, in addition, carbohydrate addiction[34].

Yes, gluten is addictive. People get addicted to bread and pasta (wheat), beer (barley), whisky or vodka (rye). On the other hand, we have never heard of the same addiction to rice, quinoa, buckwheat (not a wheat) or other non-gluten grains.

We know that most addictive substances mess with an individual's intestines and, by causing an intestinal inflammation and hampering nutrient absorption, with their brains. This addiction factor is where I see an indirect, but strong link between gluten-sensitivity and those at risk of developing type 2 diabetes.

In summary, glutens (*gluten, glutenin, gliadin*) are grain proteins present in wheat, barley, rye, spelt, triticale and, due to contamination, potentially also in oats, as well as in all their derivatives. In today's processed-food crazy world, gluten is widely used in a variety of foods because of its ability to improve texture and taste.

The "Hidden" Dangers

Never has any society consumed as much gluten as we consume today. Even more problematic than the obvious gluten content are the "hidden" glutens.

Gluten surfaces in just about all flour-products, but also in drinks, dressings, and meats (sausages, deli cuts). Even unlikely items such as ketchup, or any other products that

---

34 Nature. 2008 Nov 27;456(7221):534-8

require a "creamy" texture, may contain hidden gluten. Labels listing "natural flavors" usually indicate the presence of gluten.

In addition, gluten shows up as an undeclared carrier in two-thirds of all prescription and non-prescription medication. Many medications, thus, must be suspected for "hidden" gluten content—although they may be officially declared as "wheat free"[35].

At present, the FDA does not require gluten to be declared in prescription medications. Even in foods, the FDA's declaration policy of gluten is spotty at best because it counts as a "natural" ingredient. The bottom line is: the FDA recognizes gluten as GRAS (generally recognized as safe) and, therefore, does not bother specifying its presence.

Many potential sources of gluten contamination are not obvious. Apart from foods, these sources include items from cosmetic and personal care products to tea bags and the glue strip on envelopes.

In summary, these hidden glutens pose a huge risk to those genetically predisposed by affecting their immune system and compromising their mucosal linings (intestines, sinuses, etc.).

Carbohydrate Addiction

Glutens may hold the very key to carbohydrate addiction. Carbohydrate addiction is becoming increasingly common. Mostly, we attribute its "comfort food craving" effect to its impact on blood sugar. However, what if there was a very different explanation of the grain addiction factor? one that might look at certain grain carbohydrates as acting similar to "drugs"?

---

35 2008 CEU seminar by the American Society of Health-System Pharmacists in conjunction with the National Foundation for Celiac Awareness.

As we have seen, many of the most common grains contain gluten. Every gluten protein (similar to casein in lactose) contains small amounts of opioid-like gluten exorphins (A4, A5, B4, B5, C[36]). Their presence may explain why wheat and other gluten-containing grains can be so addictive. These proteins mimic the effect of opium in the brain.

These gluten exorphins are involved with celiac disease, diabetes, and are increasingly suspected to play a major role in many autoimmune diseases (rheumatoid arthritis, lupus, etc., diseases that recently have been spreading exponentially). Avoiding these opioid-containing glutens might also hold the key to controlling or reversing a variety of other conditions such as autism, ADD, ADHD, and behavioral problems such as aggression.

Carb Addiction Requires "Drug Detox" Approach

Comfort foods, truly, are no comfort to those who carry one of the relevant genetic factors (HLA-DQ2, DQ8, etc.). Like for an alcoholic, there is no "cure" for a "grain-carb addict." However, the accepted recommendation affords a largely symptom-free life: complete avoidance of all gluten for those who "are not born to digest grain."

There is an interesting parallel between those who recover from drug abuse and those whose body cannot handle gluten: To heal from the gluten-induced damage to the intestines, the intestines of a gluten-sensitive individual may take up to five years of a 100% gluten-free lifestyle—similar to the length of time it takes the gastrointestinal tract of a drug addict to heal.

---

36 FEBS Lett. 1992 Jan 13;296(1):107-11.

A Matter of the Gut

In individuals genetically predisposed, these gluten proteins cause damage to the intestinal lining. They mostly affect the small intestines that follow the stomach called the duodenum and the jejunum.

The numbers of those suffering from gastro-intestinal illnesses are up. A diagnosis of IBS or Crohn's should always be double-checked against the possibility of an underlying gluten-sensitivity[37], celiac disease and, potentially, a future risk of diabetes.

The Key Role of the Duodenum

The duodenum determines how much food is being released from the stomach and when. It also influences insulin, pancreatic enzymes, and liver responses along with the bile release from the gallbladder. Vitamin K production too largely depends on the duodenum.

The body's metabolism malfunctions if the duodenum becomes inflamed and is unable to digest incompatible grain proteins. Bariatric surgery results may indirectly confirm this link between duodenum, gluten-grains and diabetes:

Up to ninety-five percent of patients become free of diabetes after they undergo the Roux-en-Y gastric bypass surgery, which bypasses part of the stomach, the duodenum, and a section of the jejunum.

This is what takes place after gastric bypass surgery: Without the gluten-containing grain-carbs coming in contact with the intestinal lining, there may be no inflammation in the duodenum nor will there be change to its functions. The body's

---

37 Am J Gastroenterol. 2000 Aug;95(8):1974-82

pancreatic and liver responses can no longer misfire. Digestion and nutrient absorption are not being disturbed. As a result, the blood sugar levels stabilize.

We know that, no matter what, the diet must be changed after gastric bypass surgery—drastically. The lesson, therefore, ought to be that changing the diet may eliminate the need for surgery.

So, why not change before things go wrong? Many of these prime candidates for obesity and blood sugar fluctuations, can largely reduce and avoid intestinal inflammation and many of its resulting issues by eliminating high-carbohydrate[38], gluten-containing foods.

One must but wonder if that grain—duodenum--diabetes connection might hold the very key to reducing the future diabetes risk of many individuals worldwide[39].

Back Issues and Diabetes?

There may yet be other components to this gluten–duodenum—diabetes link. Many pre-diabetics and diabetics complain about low back pain[40] and shortness of breath.

No, it is not the weight of the beer belly that tugs on the anterior lower spine (not unlike the womb of a pregnant woman) that may affect the spinal curvature along with the body's balance. A more likely explanation involves the inflammation of the duodenum.

We have seen that a large percentage of our population experiences gut problems (bloating, loose stools, diarrhea, or

---

38 Med Hypotheses. 2006;67(2):280-2. Epub 2006 Apr 17.

39 Med Hypotheses. 2008;70(6):1207-9. Epub 2008 Feb 4; Pediatr Diabetes. 2008 Jul 28;9(4 Pt 1):335-7

40 Clin Rheumatol. 2005 Feb;24(1):76-8. Epub 2004 Sep 2.

constipation). An inflamed gut may aggravate its attachment sites (for instance to the diaphragm or the anterior lumbar spine—e.g. *ligament of Treitz*).

Manual practitioners are well aware that an inflamed duodenum may not be able to absorb the necessary minerals. This may result in body tissues and ligaments becoming rigid and brittle.

In turn, this affects the supporting ligaments and, in the case of the duodenum, the attachment to the anterior lumbar spine.

Patients who require repeated sacroiliac alignments in chiropractic or osteopathic care (particularly right-sided[41]), therefore, should always be checked for possible carbohydrate and gluten related problems[42].

Tooth Issues, Diabetes and Celiac Disease

Teeth too may be indicators of an HLA-DQ2 or HLA-DQ8 link, possible celiac disease and a risk of developing diabetes[43].

Tooth discoloration, soft teeth, loss of enamel, unusually pointed incisors, and several other dental problems have been recognized as possible early risk indicators for celiac disease.

Since carbohydrate digestion starts with the mouth, it is easy to envision that deficiencies in the oral mucosa may impact the way our body handles food in the digestive tract. Gum and tooth conditions already have been acknowledged as clear indicators of an increased diabetes risk.

---

41 Schweiz Med Wochenschr. 1979 Jul 14;109(28):1035-40

42 Dig Dis Sci. 1995 Sep;40(9):1906-8.

43 Acta Paediatr Suppl. 1996 May;412:47-8.

Mineral Deficiencies

Wherever the intestines are inflamed, absorption is compromised. Mineral deficiencies, therefore, are a common problem for diabetics and celiac disease patients alike[44].

Even long before serious disease, cravings are direct indicators of metabolic problems and of deficiencies: "Those who crave, lack."

Processed foods high in gluten-containing grains, fat and salt leave the body malnourished. But, as we have seen, deficiencies also result from lack of absorption. The practice of supplementing (often with synthetic equivalents of the missing nutrients), therefore, rarely achieves its goals.

Mineral and nutrient deficiencies directly result in increased tissue acidity, cause blood sugar spikes, and reduce the oxygen carrying ability of the blood. This is not only a vicious cycle but the beginning of an avalanche that threatens to result in a total system crash.

Already, research data indicate that a gluten-free diet in combined celiac and type 1 diabetes patients may be able to reverse bone mineral loss[45].

It is time to make that connection between grain carbohydrates (with their opioid-containing gluten content) and inflammation, between inflammation and function disturbances, between loss of regulation and diabetes.

Advocacy and Awareness Topics

I propose to raise awareness—in the medical community and the general public—about the following factors:

---

44 Eur J Gastroenterol Hepatol. 2003 Aug;15(8):851-6.

45 Pediatr Diabetes. 2008 Jul 28;9(4 Pt 1):277-84. Epub 2008 May 7

❑ A future risk of diabetes can be recognized 8 to 14 years before blood sugar levels go out of control.

❑ Over 50 health conditions and symptoms help identify that future risk of diabetes.

Further that…

❑ Diabetes may be a direct result of diet and lifestyle, however…

❑ Diabetes is largely avoidable, naturally and without costly medication, by diet and lifestyle.

And lastly that…

❑ Roughly half of our population is of the HLA-DQ2 or HLA-DQ8 genetic type.

❑ These HLA-DQ2 or HLA-DQ8 and other individuals may not be able to digest gluten grains, however, they can live a largely disease-free life by avoiding wheat, barley, rye, spelt, triticale, oats and all their derivatives.

The "Reduce Risk Lifestyle"

Rethinking Food Habits

The information is widely available.

It should not take this long for it to sicker down to the individual doctor's offices, educator desks and individuals at risk of pre-diabetes and diabetes.

Prevention must start long before the pre-diabetes stage in order to be truly effective.

Impossible? Not really, but we must focus on the recognized triggers of our epidemic diabetes numbers:

Unreasonable eating habits
❑ mostly promoted by our food industry and by our misguided and mostly outdated one-glove-fits-all diet recommendations.

Genetic predisposition
❑ that does not allow an individual to digest grain-carbohydrates without developing inflammation and subsequent system shut-down leading to immune system or metabolic disease such as diabetes.

Overfed and Malnourished

Unreasonable eating habits along with a genetic predisposition make for a high risk of metabolic disease and diabetes.

Never has the lack of nutrients played so much havoc with human nature. World hunger is an issue, but never has the WHO estimated so many overfed, malnourished people[46].

Starting with many of our heavily promoted food pyramids, including the Standard American Diet (S.A.D.), those individuals at risk of diabetes will have to distance themselves from decades of in-"grained" food habits.

We cannot avoid or control diabetes by starting the day with a veritable sugar-bonanza consisting of orange juice, corn flakes or any other form of grain cereals and milk—all foods that convert to sugar in the body.

The Bottom Line

For effective avoidance, control or reversal of diabetes, research points to the need to greater selfcare.

- Mindless food choices rob the body's new cells of their potential.

- Thoughtful food choices allow the body's new cells to develop their full potential.

---

46 http://www.who.int/nutrition/topics/obesity/en/index.html

Avoid

- ❏ high-carbohydrate, starchy foods (grains and starchy vegetables)
- ❏ processed foods
- ❏ trans fat and other solid fat containing foods
- ❏ foods high in sodium (processed foods contain twenty times more salt than our daily requirement)
- ❏ beer and other alcoholic beverages (they are high in sugar and high in nutrient-poor calories)
- ❏ soft drinks (diet or otherwise)
- ❏ sugars in any form (that includes anything ending in – ose)
- ❏ preservatives including salt, nitrates, sodium benzoate, etc.
- ❏ colors
- ❏ flavors ("natural" flavors include gluten)
- ❏ other additives
- ❏ smoking
- ❏ use of drugs
- ❏ physical inactivity.

These recommendations are not only part of the avoid-list for a risk of diabetes. They should become the avoid-list for any disease and for a healthy overall lifestyle.

On the other hand, the research recommendations for a healthy lifestyle, effective avoidance, control or reversal of diabetes and many other conditions, point to the following measures to favor.

Favor

- ❑ loads of green and colorful, non-starchy vegetables
- ❑ Berries and low-sugar, high-antioxidant fruit
- ❑ Fish, light meats (chicken, turkey and other fowl, game) and eggs (from chickens free of antibiotic feed)
- ❑ Olive and grapeseed oils
- ❑ Ample fresh, non-chlorinated water
- ❑ Green and other antioxidant teas
- ❑ Daily physical activity.

In Summary

The logic is straight forward:

- ❑ The body replaces some of its cells continuously.
- ❑ The average lifetime of a cell lasts from 105 to 125 days.
- ❑ Therefore, every morsel of food that goes into the mouth, directly affects the newly developing cells.

The body's ageing and disease processes exactly and directly reflect the way we eat at the time these cells develop.

Depending on our genetic background, there are certain food groups that our body is not equipped to handle.

By increasing public knowledge and awareness about these physiological processes, we can equip the individual to live according to these facts.

We would never think of putting diesel into the tank of a gas-driven car. We must learn not to put incompatible grain-carbohydrates into the system of individuals whose body is not equipped to handle them.

NOTES:

Author Bio

Rivkah Roth DO DNM® is a natural medicine professional, lecturer, and author with doctorates in osteopathy, natural medicine, acupuncture and traditional Chinese medicine. She is also the author of "At Risk? Avoid Diabetes by Recognizing Early Risk – A Natural Medicine View" and the DIABETES-Series Little Books.

Over the decades, Rivkah Roth has lectured in Canada, Switzerland, and the Middle East and has won awards and accolades for her dedication and contribution to the field of natural medicine. She lives, writes, and practices in Ontario, Canada, from where she offers web-based support programs for the general public and advanced training seminars for health professionals. In-person or Skype consultations are available by appointment only. Visit her at www.avoidiabetes.com

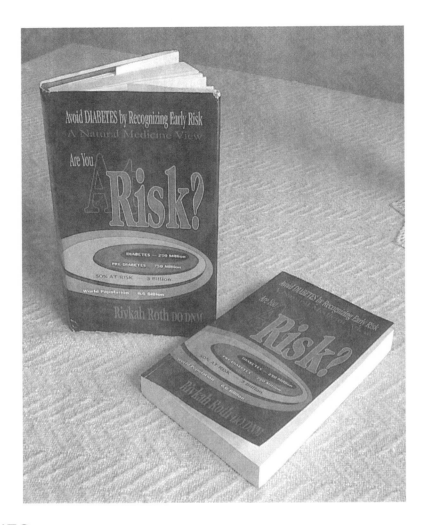

INFO

At Risk? Avoid DIABETES by Recognizing Early Risk – A Natural Medicine View
(All-in-one volume contains text, "FACT" Summary, recommendations and workbook pages)

Second Edition 2009 - 396 pages – 20 Graphs and Illustrations
ISBN 1-978-0-9812297-0-6

First Edition 2008:
Library of Congress Control Number 2008905554
Cloth Hardcover ISBN 978-1-4257-6174-5
Trade Paperback ISBN 978-1-4257-6169-1

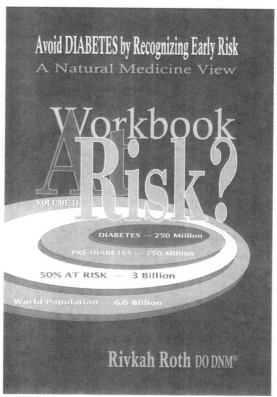

INFO

At Risk? Expanded Workbook
> *Avoid DIABETES by Recognizing Early Risk*
> *– A Natural Medicine View*
> Expanded Workbook, "FACT" Summary and
> Recommendations
> Softcover ISBN 978-1-981-2297-9-9

NATURAL MEDICINE CENTRE – PUBLISHING
Toronto

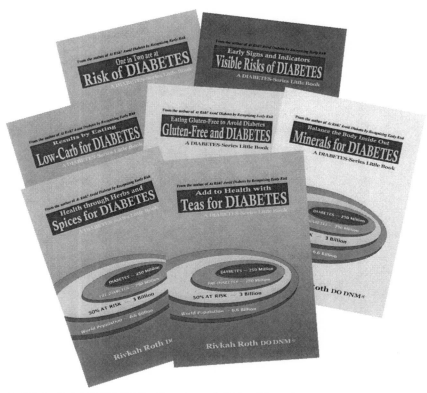

INFO DIABETES-Series Little Books

1-topic, point-form, easy to read, 48-page titles

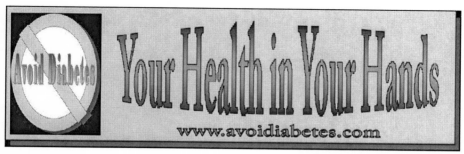

info@avoidiabetes.com

Natural Medicine Support

for the At-Risk, Pre-Diabetes & Diabetes Patient

❑ Early Diabetes Risk Assessment
❑ Natural Lifestyle and Nutritional Assessments & Support
❑ Natural Medicine Support to Avoid, Control and Reverse Diabetes and its Complications

Webinar Series
Scheduled Online Q & A Sessions
Group and Individual Consults

"At Risk?" - "Reduce Your Risk!"

Specialization Training
for the HEALTH PROFESSIONAL
Who wants to make a difference in the lives of many more patients

❑ Certification Programs & Upgrade Courses
❑ Professional Support Seminars

GET HELP if you need it!
Diabetes is largely Avoidable
HELP if you can!

CPSIA information can be obtained at www.ICGtesting.com
Printed in the USA
BVOW09s1019240214

345830BV00002B/285/P